RATIONING OF HEALTH AND SOCIAL CARE

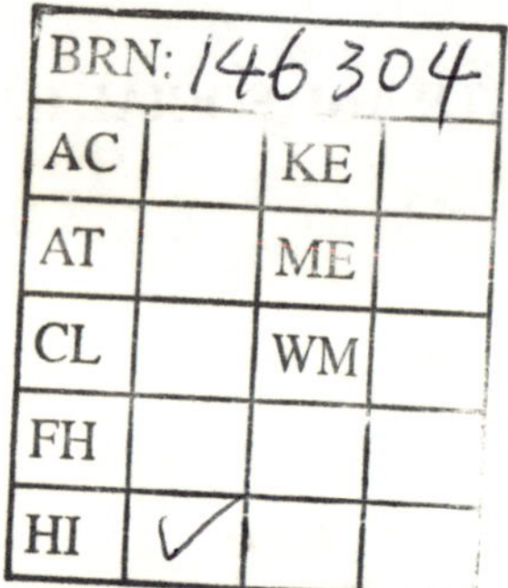

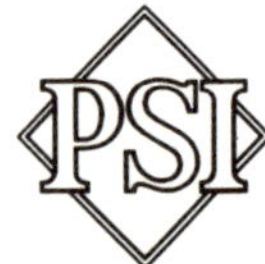

The Policy Studies Institute (PSI) is Britain's leading independent research organisation undertaking studies of economic, industrial and social policy, and the workings of political institutions.

PSI is a registered charity, run on a non-profit basis, and is not associated with any political party, pressure group or commercial interest.

PSI attaches great importance to covering a wide range of subject areas with its multi-disciplinary approach. The Institute's 40+ researchers are organised in teams which currently cover the following programmes:

Family Finances – Employment – Information Policy – Social Justice and Social Order – Health Studies and Social Care – Education – Industrial Policy and Futures – Arts and the Cultural Industries – Environment and Quality of Life

This publication arises from the Social Care and Health Studies programme and is one of over 30 publications made available by the Institute each year.

Information about the work of PSI, and a catalogue of available books can be obtained from:

Marketing Department, PSI
100 Park Village East, London NW1 3SR

Other ADSS Conference Papers available from PSI

DRAWING THE LINE: Purchasing and Providing Social Services in the 1990s £7.95 (1991)

HEALTH AND SOCIAL SERVICES: The New Relationship £7.95 (1990)

CARE MANAGERS AND CARE MANAGEMENT £7.95 (1989)

Rationing of Health and Social Care

Edited by Isobel Allen

The ADSS/PSI Group is supported by the Joseph Rowntree Foundation

Policy Studies Institute, London

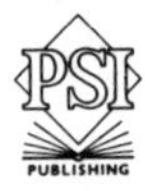

The publishing imprint of the independent
POLICY STUDIES INSTITUTE
100 Park Village East, London NW1 3SR
Telephone: 071-387 2171 Fax: 071-388 0914

ISBN 0 85374 583 8

PSI Research Report 757

A CIP catalogue record of this book is available from the British Library.

1 2 3 4 5 6 7 8 9

PSI publications are available from
BEBC Distribution Ltd
P O Box 1496, Poole, Dorset, BH12 3YD

Books will normally be despatched within 24 hours. Cheques should be made payable to BEBC Distribution Ltd.

Credit card and telephone/fax orders may be placed on the following freephone numbers:

FREEPHONE: 0800 262260
FREEFAX: 0800 262266

PSI subscriptions are available from PSI's subscription agent
Carfax Publishing Company Ltd
P O Box 25, Abingdon, Oxford OX14 3UE

Laserset by Policy Studies Institute
Printed in Great Britain by BPCC Wheatons Ltd, Exeter

Contents

Preface

This Discussion Paper brings together the papers delivered at the annual seminar held by the Association of Directors of Social Services (ADSS) and Policy Studies Institute (PSI) in November 1992. The theme of the seminar was ***Rationing of Health and Social Care.***

The question of how far it is possible to satisfy need when resources are finite is a central issue in health and social care provision. A system of rationing has always been applied to the provision of services, but much of this rationing has often been implicit rather than explicit. However, there is growing recognition that rationing of both health and social care is not only becoming more explicit but also that guidelines may be needed to determine the level and type of such rationing.

The seminar started by examining experience in the health service where the debate has already been opened up in a number of countries. Two perspectives were presented by Professor Chris Ham, Health Services Management Centre, University of Birmingham, and John James, District General Manager of Parkside District Health Authority.

We then looked more closely at practical experience at a local level with a joint paper from Joyce Moseley, Director of Social Services, London Borough of Hackney, and Dr Bobbie Jacobson, Director of Public Health, City and Hackney District Health Authority, describing how social services and health authorities are working together in Hackney to tackle the problems of needs assessment and provision of services.

The final session examined some of the ethical and philosophical issues which arise when rationing of health and social care have to be tackled by policy-makers and managers alike. Terry Bamford, Executive Director of Housing and Social Services, Royal Borough of Kensington and Chelsea, reflected on the practical questions involved in deciding who gets what, when and in what volume, while Jeff Girling, Senior Fellow at the Health Services Management Unit, University of Manchester, presented a paper examining the ethical framework in which managers make their decisions.

The aim of the seminars organised by the Association of Directors of Social Services and Policy Studies Institute is to stimulate debate among practitioners, researchers and policy-makers on the most topical issues in social policy. The seminars are supported by a grant from the Joseph Rowntree Foundation.

Isobel Allen
Policy Studies Institute

Priority Setting in the Health Services: Lessons from Experience

Professor Chris Ham
Health Services Management Centre, University of Birmingham

Priority setting is neither new to the NHS nor unique to the UK. Within the NHS, there has always been a process of priority setting and rationing, the most manifest example being the existence of waiting lists for some treatments. Outside the UK, several countries have shown an interest in adopting a more systematic approach to setting priorities. These include the Netherlands, New Zealand, Sweden, and the state of Oregon in the United States. What is different about the present position is that priority setting is becoming more difficult.

There are a number of reasons for this. To begin with, developments in medical technology are making it possible to undertake more investigations and to provide additional services. In parallel, the ageing population has resulted in extra demands being placed on health services. The resources allocated to the NHS have continued to grow but there is an increasing gap between what it is possible to do as a result of medical advances and what it is possible to fund with the available budget. It is for this reason that priority setting presents an increasingly difficult challenge for policy makers.

Another new factor to take into account is the impact of the NHS reforms. A central element within the reforms is the separation of responsibility for purchasing and providing health services. District health authorities as purchasers are in the position of having to determine local priorities for service developments. In their purchasing role, health authorities have to establish more explicit priorities and to translate these into contracts with providers. This means that priority setting will in future will be less covert than in the past and health authorities will have to defend their decisions on which services should receive additional resources and which should receive lower priority.

All the evidence suggests that district health authorities will have the main responsibility for priority setting. At a national level, the Department of Health has set three major national priorities. These are to improve the health of the nation through the national health strategy; to raise the quality of health services through the Patient's Charter; and to implement the reforms to community care. In addition, a high priority has been attached to shifting resources towards primary care and away from secondary care services.

There are some real tensions within these national priorities. The most obvious is that between the concern for individual rights and collective responsibility. Health authorities in their purchasing role have to balance a range of demands and needs. As such, they are responsible for taking a population-wide view of health services and establishing some clear priorities for the improvement of health. At the same time, the Patient's Charter is encouraging individual patients to be more assertive in their use of services and to have higher expectations of the quality of care. Health authorities cannot always respond positively to individual demands and they have to make an overall judgement about what is in the community's interest as a whole.

The dilemma here is well illustrated by the case of Laura Davies. Laura is the little girl who became seriously ill and required a combined bowel and liver transplant. This operation is not currently available in the UK and she travelled to the United States to undergo treatment at the transplant centre there that is at the forefront of the development of this particular service. Health authorities have to decide the priority they are prepared to give to this kind of treatment, involving expenditure of around £300,000 in Laura's case, compared with the priority to be given to other services. If you consider the number of hip replacement or cataract operations that could be bought for £300,000, and the questions that have been raised about the long-term benefits of this kind of innovative treatment, it is easy to see how health authorities have to make some very difficult choices. The point that is important here is that it is the population-wide view that health authorities must take into account and they cannot respond positively to the demands of all individuals – difficult as this may be.

Local experience

In recognition of the key role of health authorities in setting priorities, I undertook a piece of work last year in the Southampton and South West Hampshire Health Authority. The work involved a simulation with the Health Authority of some of the issues involved in priority setting. The Health Authority took 24 hours 'time out' to work through three cases: coronary heart disease, the treatment of elderly people following a stroke, and the balance of spending between different care groups. The result of this work was published in a King's Fund College paper, *Purchasing Dilemmas*, published earlier this year (Heginbotham and Ham, 1992).

Before drawing out the lessons of the Southampton work I would like to indicate the way in which we summarised the role of the health authority in the Southampton simulation. Figure 1 illustrates the position of the health authority in responding to competing pressures and demands.

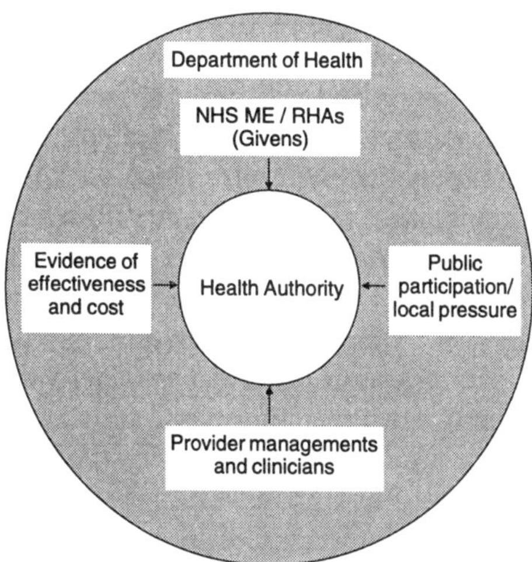

The vertical axis represents the main sources of pressure on health authorities in the past. At one level, there are the national and regional pressures resulting from the priorities set by health ministers and regional health authorities. District health authorities have little choice but to respond to these pressures and to adapt them to suit local circumstances. At another level, there are the views of local providers and professionals. It is these views that have often been most important when health authorities have made their decisions. Professional priorities have been given considerable importance in the NHS in the past and health authorities have been dominated by the views of professionals in their decision making.

The opportunity created by the NHS reforms is for the pressures on the horizontal axis to be given greater emphasis. Ministers are fond of talking of district health authorities as being 'champions of the people'. On the face of it, this description has little credibility, given the current composition of health authorities. Nevertheless, the idea is important in highlighting the potential role of health authorities in using their purchasing power to achieve a better fit between the population's need for health care and the use of resources.

If they are to be credible champions of the people, health authorities must find ways of involving the local community in decision making. This is already happening in many parts of the country. District health authorities are experimenting with various techniques and methods of engaging with the public and encouraging local participation. Many of the results of this work were summarised in the Department of Health's report, *Local Voices*, published in 1991.

Alongside the views of local people, health authorities are increasingly examining evidence on the cost effectiveness of different services in deciding what to purchase. This is the other side of the horizontal axis. In the past, when decisions were strongly influenced by the views of local providers and professionals, evidence on cost effectiveness did not figure strongly in the decision-making process. Now that health authorities are purchasers of health care and responsibility for service provision rests increasingly with NHS trusts, there is a better basis for health authorities to take a more questioning view of some of the claims made by professional groups. In so doing, they are increasingly making use of data produced by health economists and epidemiologists in determining what local priorities should be.

Turning to the Southampton simulation, a number of important lessons and conclusions emerged. First, we quickly discovered that information on costs and benefits was incomplete. This meant that health authorities had to take their decisions in conditions of considerable uncertainty.

Second, priority setting cannot be reduced to a technical exercise. This is sometimes the claim made by health economists when they refer to the use of QALY league tables and suggest that the cost effectiveness data represented by QALY league tables should help to determine decision making. The reality is that, given the incompleteness of information, health authorities have to use more than simply scientific evidence in arriving at priority decisions.

Third, following on from this, health authorities cannot escape making judgements in discussing priorities. It is impossible to determine the relative balance of spending between different care groups on the basis of data alone. These decisions are inherently value judgements which are best made by a group of lay people properly informed by evidence and the views of professionals. In this sense, decision making on priorities is a matter of debate and argument in which health authorities should provide a lead.

Fourth, in Southampton we found that the most difficult choices are those about the relative priority to be attached to different care groups. This is because these choices involve comparisons between quite different services. It was somewhat easier to look at the balance of spending within individual care group or disease group categories. For example, in looking at coronary heart disease, the health authority made more progress in discussing the balance between prevention, treatment, and other options for addressing coronary heart disease, than it did when it came to looking at the overall distribution of the budget between the full range of services.

Fifth, the Southampton work confirmed the importance of there being a public debate about priority setting. Health authorities have to be able to defend the decisions they make. This is easier done if the process that has led up to those decisions is open and accessible. However, as many health authorities have discovered, engaging with the public in a debate about priorities is difficult. Health authorities have to be imaginative in finding more effective ways of stimulating local discussion.

Questions about priority setting

Looking beyond the Southampton experience, a number of key questions have arisen as the debate about priority setting in the NHS has evolved. One important issue is whether health authorities should seek to exclude certain services altogether. The examples often mentioned in debate are *in vitro* fertilisation, tattoo removal, treatment of varicose veins, and reversal of sterilisation.

My own view is that this path is not particularly promising. The reality is that in all of these cases it can be argued that some patients need the interventions concerned and are able to benefit from them. There are very few services provided within the NHS which ought to be excluded entirely. In practice, as Rudolf Klein's recent work has shown, on the whole health authorities have avoided making exclusions and have concentrated on more incremental approaches to priority setting (Klein and Redmayne, 1992).

A second issue is the role of the health authority in setting priorities in relation to the role of doctors. It is clear that both GPs and consultants will continue to play a major part in determining priorities. This applies especially when it comes to determining which particular patients should receive treatment and at what point. Yet at the same time, health authorities are in a position of having to take more explicit decisions on priorities for the use of their resources. In the Southampton work, this arose as a particular concern, not least in the health authority avoiding being too prescriptive in its decisions and leaving no room for discretion by clinicians. A delicate balance has to be struck here.

A third issue is the role of clinical guidelines and protocols. There is increasing interest in the development of guidelines and protocols throughout the NHS. In essence, guidelines seek to establish a framework within which GPs and consultants can deliver services. They vary in their level of detail but an essential contribution of guidelines is to specify which patients with which conditions are most likely to benefit from treatment. Considerable effort has been put into developing guidelines for the treatment of common conditions such as asthma and diabetes, and there is a role for them in a range of other areas too. Again, my own view based on experience is that this is a particularly promising way forward, and that at a local level, doctors and managers need to be adapting the guidelines which have been established nationally to suit their own purposes.

Conclusion

Let me make a number of concluding comments. To begin with, I think it is important to recognise the different levels of rationing. At a minimum, rationing involves decisions at a national, local and individual level. There is therefore a role for the Department of Health, health authorities and health care professionals. None has an exclusive preserve on decisions in this area.

It is also important to recognise the need to combine techniques with debate. If priority setting cannot be reduced to a technical cum scientific process, ways have to be found of stimulating local debate and discussion of priority setting. In this sense, the horizontal axis of the Southampton simulation figure is the important one on which to focus. Evidence on costs and effectiveness needs to be combined with the gathering of local views and opinions in order to help health authorities make sensible decisions on priorities.

Another important conclusion is that rationing should be looked at in terms of 'bite-sized chunks'. As I mentioned earlier, the most difficult decisions are those involving comparisons between quite different services and care groups. In the short term, it is more likely that progress can be made by identifying specific service areas and reviewing the balance of spending within these service areas. Incremental decisions of this kind seem to me to offer the most promising way forward in the immediate future.

Finally, the evidence suggests that even simple approaches to priority setting can be helpful. I am currently doing some work on behalf of the NHS Management Executive Research and Development Directorate reviewing the experience of six health authorities in priority setting. One of the conclusions coming out of this is that a range of different approaches and techniques are being used around the NHS. It is unrealistic to expect health authorities in the UK to emulate Oregon and set up an extensive and expensive ranking exercise. Much more likely is that health authorities will pursue modest approaches in their own districts to adopt a more systematic approach than has hitherto been the case. It is in this context that simple and relatively crude approaches have a part to play.

References

Heginbotham, C. and Ham, C. (1992), *Purchasing Dilemmas*, King's Fund College, London.

Klein, R. and Redmayne, S. (1992), *Patterns of Priorities*, NAHAT, Birmingham.

Health Care Rationing: Lessons from a District Health Authority

John H. James
District General Manager, Parkside District Health Authority

The topic of health care rationing is not in any sense new but has come more and more out of the closet in recent years. This analysis falls into two parts. First it suggests a general framework for thinking about rationing of health care. Secondly it describes the results of real life experiments conducted within my District Health Authority. I should say by way of parenthesis that for eighteen months I managed two District Health Authorities simultaneously, and I was therefore fortunate enough to be able to try out ideas in two different locations.

It is possible to see the way in which rationing in health care has gone on in this country as a process of evolution. Before the introduction of the NHS, access to health care depended on having the means to pay or being fortunate enough to be able to take advantage of charitable or local authority facilities. The NHS created universal access, free at the point of use, even though from a relatively early stage prescription charges operated both as a means of raising revenue and as an intended deterrent. The NHS's architects thought that the system would in time become less expensive as the overall health of the nation improved, an expectation which was quickly disappointed. Successive attempts were made over many years to hold down the rising costs. Curiously little attention was paid until the 1970s to the fact that every other developed country was also experiencing rising costs. Rationing nonetheless was essentially done, and far more efficiently here than anywhere else, by limiting the total amount of money that went into the system. Finite resources were then matched with demand largely at the level of the individual clinician. Decisions to treat and decisions on urgency were taken by the consultant. The waiting list acted as a safety valve. The GP would judge whether to make a hospital referral by reference to waiting times. By and large emergencies were well handled, the elective end of the work was not.

The process of challenging this implicit rationing took a long time. The neglected back wards of the long stay mental illness and mental handicap hospitals had been an easy target for savings, but enquiries into major scandals at Ely and Whittingham hospitals in the late 1960s presaged a deliberate decision to give increased priority to the so-called Cinderella services. Services for the elderly followed. The acute sector came to be seen as an undue consumer of resources.

Challenges to rationing *within* the acute sector can be detected from the early 1980s onwards. Limitation on access to the end-stage renal failure treatment programmes was one area of pressure. The Secretary of State at the time, Norman Fowler, responded by setting targets for levels of intervention which were quickly followed by others such as hip replacements and coronary artery bypass grafts. A more serious challenge came as a result of the apparent failure of Birmingham Children's Hospital to find a bed for a four year old child requiring heart surgery. This episode, together with a general perception that underfunding lay at the heart of the NHS's inability to keep pace with demand for acute health care, ultimately led to the Government's 1989 NHS reforms in the White Paper, *Working for Patients.*

At the heart of the reforms, although its significance was not immediately appreciated, lay an assumption that in future it would not be the clinician alone who determined rationing priorities, but that the responsibility would be laid primarily on the purchasers of health care. The District Health Authorities and the general practice fundholders, who were given budgets in order to purchase health care for a given population, had expressly to consider, and agree with a range of hospitals and other providers, how much health care they could afford to buy. Thus in the current year, Parkside Health Authority has contracted in total for some 80,000 episodes of acute health care. This will cover in patient and day care. Contracts have been placed with some 20 acute hospitals, each defining an expected number of episodes, albeit with a 5 per cent tolerance either way. At an aggregate level therefore the Authority has taken responsibility for overall rationing decisions. Indicative numbers of cases within particular specialties have also been agreed. Thus the Authority has bought a finite number of, for example, orthopaedic episodes. The contracts may well also specify in quite an amount of detail the expected case complexity. The rationing is therefore explicit. Indeed already two of the Authority's major providing hospitals are substantially exceeding the contracted activity levels, and both are obliged to restrict admissions to emergencies in the last quarter of the year in order to stay within the contracted levels. There is of course nothing very new about this. Hospitals have customarily closed parts of their facilities in order to stay within budget. What is different this year is that the hospital may, in some cases, question the judgement of the purchaser in not placing a sufficiently large contract. In other words it is challenging the purchaser's decisions on rationing.

This state of affairs was foreseeable, and it is equally possible to see that next year will be more difficult still. How then does the Health Authority put itself into a position whereby it can justify the rationing decisions it has taken? Broadly speaking, the approach best adopted has been to work very closely with general practitioners, to identify their priorities and preferences, to develop and consult upon purchasing intentions, concentrating on changes, and to seek to develop a public debate, which will widen the legitimacy both of the values that are adopted, and of the explicit decisions that are taken, beyond the immediate confines of the Health Authority. The use of health needs assessment to improve our understanding of health need in the population, use and dispersion of the steadily improving flow of information about the effectiveness of different forms of clinical intervention, together with the cost, particularly where they differ between different hospitals – all of these are part of the legitimate weapons of opening up the debate. Most GPs, it seems, are influenced by knowledge of relative costs. Parkside Health Authority published a GP handbook in each of the last two years giving relative costs, and many GPs have told us that it has influenced their referring practice. Harrow GPs have emphasised the same point, although there was concern when we decided to end our contract with the Royal National Orthopaedic Hospital because it was significantly more expensive for day to day work than the other four local hospitals which did orthopaedic work. The concern centred on the principle of choice. The DHA's reaction was that it would always look at any case on its merits, but at the end of the day a decision to refer a patient to a particular hospital at twice the price of an alternative freely available locally is an implicit decision to deny treatment to one or more *other* people. Choice has its price.

Before the realities of rationing hit, it was decided to give the members of both Parkside and Harrow Health Authorities – executive and non-executive – some dry run opportunities to think through the issues. Thus in the earlier part of last year each member was asked individually to rank ten different aspects of health care in priority order. Most, even the non-executives, placed, for example, resettlement of mentally ill people higher than heart transplants, showing that they were using a values framework which placed quality of life above the avoidance of death. Each member was also asked to place a series of values in priority order. These included aspects such as adding life to years or years to life, equity between different ethnic groups, local accessibility and so on. Interestingly, Harrow gave a low rating to adding years to life, whereas Parkside placed it second to adding life to years. The results of the values judgement were then built into mission statements for both Authorities.

More elaborate experiments followed and were linked to the decisions which the two Authorities would have to take on priorities for investment in 1992-93. In both cases, although the Authorities received no growth, they had made savings in their traditional acute contracts in order to create a development pool. Each had a list of potential investments that it could make, and the exercise was part of the decision making process. It was not however the entire basis of the process, since the possible development proposals were selected at random from a larger number.

For Parkside (Figure 1) six proposals were examined – additional investment in renal services, a new community-based mental illness team covering part of Brent, increased open access physiotherapy, expanded rehabilitation services, additional nursing home places, and funding of a voluntary body to bathe old people in their own homes, where the need for bathing was social rather than clinically-based. The members were given enough detail of each proposal to know what benefits it would deliver, and what it would cost. They were then asked to use eleven criteria which had been developed by a non-executive member of Parkside DHA and to place the six developments in priority order against each of the eleven criteria. The criteria are set out in

Figure 1

Costs £000s

	1992-93	Full year
1. EXPANSION OF RENAL SERVICES Additional investment at St Mary's	700	700
2 MENTAL HEALTH COMMUNITY ASSESSMENT & SHORT-TERM SUPPORT TEAM (CASTS) 10 strong multi-disciplinary team in Brent	223	306
3 YOUNGER DISABLED LONG TERM NURSING HOME PLACEMENTS	350	350
4 SOCIAL BATHING 50% contribution to voluntary group	15	0
5 DIRECT ACCESS GP PHYSIOTHERAPY at Central Middlesex Hospital	60	100
6 REHABILITATION Surgical, neurological & community outreach (4 linked schemes)	317	407

Figure 2. In each case members were asked to rank the proposal low, medium or high against the criteria and these were translated into scores of 1, 2 or 3. Thus if a project was accorded a low value against all eleven criteria it would score a total of eleven points, with a high value it could go up to thirty-three.

At aggregate level, the exercise demonstrated a clear order of priority (Figure 3). The mental illness service came highest and social bathing came lowest. Both largely performed consistently across the criteria (Figure 4). There were, however, significant differences between individual members' perceptions of the relative importance of the projects (Figure 5). For example member number 5 accorded second highest priority to social bathing, while member number 1 placed the mental illness project only fourth out of the six.

Using the value criteria quickly demonstrated the shortcomings. They are motherhood-and-apple pie, they overlap, some of them are

Figure 2

Parkside Health Authority – Health Gain Seminar

Establishing criteria against which to prioritise health gain investment decisions. The criteria/questions which have so far emerged against which the Health Authority might test/prioritise each service investment:

1. To what extent does the proposal address significant health needs – identified through public comment, epidemiological evidence or patterns of clinical practice?
2. To what extent would the proposal contribute to promoting better health for people and preventing ill-health (i.e. by improving personal well being and reducing avoidable morbidity and mortality)?
3. To what extent will the proposal contribute to curing or ameliorating ill-health (as reflected in maintaining or restoring the capacity of people for a full life, reducing pain and discomfort, or enhancing longevity)?
4. To what extent would the proposal contribute to improving equity between different groups in health outcomes and/or in access to appropriate and sensitive services?
5. To what extent would the proposal contribute to strengthening the control local people can exercise over the conditions affecting their health and the services available to meet their health needs?
6. To what extent would the proposal increase people's access to good quality services relevant to their health needs?
7. To what extent would the proposal minimise the disruption to people's everyday lives consequent upon needing treatment or care?
8. To what extent would the proposal improve the acceptability of the way services are delivered?
9. To what extent would the proposal contribute to future improvements in the capacity of the NHS to deliver good quality health services (i.e. by contributing to scientific knowledge or attracting and developing the skills of staff)?
10. To what extent is the proposal an efficient means for delivering these gains?
11. What is the likely cost?
12. To what extent is the District likely to be able to secure effective implementation of the proposal (e.g. through the support of GPs and providers)?

David Towell

Figure 3

Proposal	Score	Position
1 Renal	224	2nd
2 CASTS	244	1st
3 Nursing homes	195	5th
4 Social bathing	180	6th
5 Physiotherapy	209	4th
6 Rehabilitation	212	3rd

Figure 4

The proposals ranked differently for the 11 criteria as follows

Proposal	Criteria	1	2	3	4	5	6	7	8	9	10	11
Renal	1	1st	2nd	1st	3rd	6th	2nd	2nd	6th	1st	2nd	2nd
Mental illness CASTS	2	2nd	1st	4th	1st	1st	1st	1st	1st	3rd	2nd	5th
Nursing homes	3	5th	6th	5th	2nd	4th	4th	6th	2nd	5th	4th	3rd
Social bathing	4	6th	4th	6th	5th	2nd	6th	4th	4th	6th	6th	6th
Open access physio	5	4th	5th	3rd	6th	3rd	5th	2nd	3rd	3rd	1st	1st
Rehab.	6	2nd	3rd	2nd	4th	4th	2nd	5th	4th	2nd	4th	3rd

multiple choice and there are too many of them. It is also arguable that they should be given different weightings. Indeed one might argue that the weightings should be influenced by a pre-selection into particular categories. Thus, for example, social bathing is not intended to meet research objectives, contribute to undergraduate teaching or to save

Figure 5 Health gain criteria – total scores

Investment proposal no.	Numbered Health Authority members												
	1	**2**	**3**	**4**	**5**	**6**	**7**	**8**	**9**	**Range**	**Mean**	**Total score**	**Pos.**
1	26	23	21	23	24	25	29	23	30	21-30	25	224	2nd
2	23	29	23	28	29	26	30	26	31	23-31	28	244	1st
3	19	17	23	23	23	25	22	18	25	17-25	22	195	5th
4	22	19	19	15	25	22	24	12	22	17-25	20	180	6th
5	25	23	24	17	22	23	26	22	27	17-26	24	209	4th
6	28	24	19	24	24	25	20	25	23	19-28	24	212	3rd
Total	143	135	129	130	147	146	153	126	158	126-158			

The table shows the score given to each proposal by each Health Authority member, the range of scoring, the mean, total score and rank.

life; but it may be vital in enabling somebody to stay at home who would otherwise be blocking a bed elsewhere. We have therefore emerged from the process better equipped to use systematic assessment criteria to determine next year's priorities. As a footnote, Parkside did indeed invest in all of the six proposals except the increased open access physiotherapy.

Apart from recognising the shortcomings of the criteria, the main lesson we derived from this particular set of exercises, was that, provided one has an explicit set of value criteria and good information on both the benefits and the costs of a particular course of action, it is possible to improve one's understanding of choice through this kind of exercise. However, it is much easier when it is a matter of deciding which of several desirable alternatives should actually be introduced. It will be much harder when it is applied to the decision what to *cease* doing. That will be the next stage.

One only has to look at the furore which surrounded the Oregon experiment to recognise the dangers and difficulties involved in rationing when it is a matter of visible restrictions of access to services which already exist. The Parkside and Harrow exercise was relatively undemanding, because it was a matter of whether to invest where investments were not presently being made. Oregon involved a much more substantial redistribution of investment, and even though the proposal would actually have led to increased expenditure, the all or nothing approach was bound to be controversial. In the United Kingdom, we are far more likely to find ourselves rationing the quantum of care within each category than trying to restrict categories. The obvious targets – varicose veins and cosmetic plastic surgery – for total bans on provision quickly evaporate when one begins to consider that there may be a proportion of cases for example of rhinoplasty that can be justified because of the psychological damage which the pre-operative condition is causing to the individuals. In practice there may be little prospect of seeking to define, by precise regulation, any exclusive criteria.

Another area which has been looked at extensively is whether to define the criteria for access to infertility treatment or to deal with it on a case-by-case basis. The argument for definition is that there is a clinically accepted set of criteria that has been adopted by most of the major centres, and as there is a reasonable degree of consistency about these, it is possible to latch on to them. That said, in what is obviously a highly charged topic, the appearance of rigid rules may create an unwillingness to cooperate with them greater than if they had been explained and applied on a case-by-case basis.

Overall the approach to rationing is still very crude and primitive in the NHS. It will have to become much less so very quickly if Health Authorities are to command confidence in the decisions that they now take more overtly than was previously the case on behalf of the general population. It remains to be seen how well we will meet the challenge to do this.

Needs Assessment and Rationing in Health and Social Care

Joyce Moseley
Director of Social Services, London Borough of Hackney

Dr Bobbie Jacobson
Director of Public Health, City & Hackney District Health Authority

Introduction (Joyce Moseley)

To show the level of our collaboration Bobbie Jacobson and I are going to set the Hackney scene in a joint paper. I will give some basic facts and figures and Bobbie Jacobson will explain our joint planning system in which our needs assessment work should take place. My part of the paper will concentrate on assessing individual need. Bobbie Jacobson will cover assessing population need and will then draw together some concluding comments.

Facts and figures about Hackney

Figure 1 shows Hackney as a small London Borough with a young population. The Census does not record ethnic minorities in a way which is adequate for needs assessment. For instance it takes no account of the Orthodox Jewish communities or the Turkish and Kurdish communities which have specific needs for both health and social care. The refugee figure is an estimate by the Public Health Department.

Figure 1 Hackney populations, 1991

	%	Number
Total population		181,248
Ethnic minorities	33.6	61,000
Under 5	8.4	15,000
Over 65	14.2	25,000
Over 85	1.1	2,000

Estimated 23,000 refugees

Figure 2 shows Hackney to be very deprived on all social and health indices. The high rate for schizophrenia is indicated in early findings of research being done presently. The quote from the District Audit Service leaves one a little daunted.

Figure 2 Deprivation indicators

- DoE assessment based on 1991 Census – most deprived borough
- Second highest Jarman score in the country
- SSA for Hackney is 25 per cent above Inner London average at £55.5m (budget over SSA by £2m)
- Death rate (15-64 year olds) 21 per cent higher than national average
- 20 per cent higher rate of schizophrenia
- Highest percentage single parents – 8.4 households
- 3rd highest overcrowding
- Highest unemployment 22 per cent (men)

'The figures are presented here to underline the contention that demand for Health and Social Care in this part of London is significantly greater than the resources available' (*District Audit, Review of Community Care*, October 1992).

Figure 3 indicates major changes and instability at a time when stability is needed if we are going to progress joint working. However, not all is gloom and doom, as Hackney is attracting investment which will improve the physical fabric. This in the long run is likely to do as much for health and social care needs as our joint services.

Figure 3 A time of change

Instability in health

- DHA merger – loss of coterminosity
- Review of primary and community health care
- Tomlinson

New resources in Hackney

- City Challenge
- Estate improvements
- Resulting from political and managerial stability

Joint working (Bobbie Jacobson)

Community care implementation has been able to rely on a strong tradition of joint working and good collaborative arrangements (see Figure 4). Those parts of the structure that still need fine tuning include the development of user and community participation mechanisms.

Needs assessment and rationing in social care at the individual level (Joyce Moseley)

Following a recent discussion with Bobbie Jacobson and a colleague from the District Audit Service, I had a flash of clarity about the inter-relationships between needs assessment of populations on the one hand and assessment of needs of individuals on the other hand, across our two services. And hands were important in the process of understanding, as there were a lot of hand movements to explain the needs assessment process. I developed this into a model that I have called The Four Spider Model (see Figure 5).

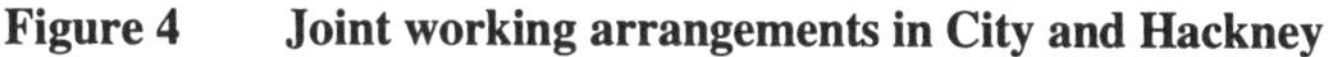

Figure 4 Joint working arrangements in City and Hackney

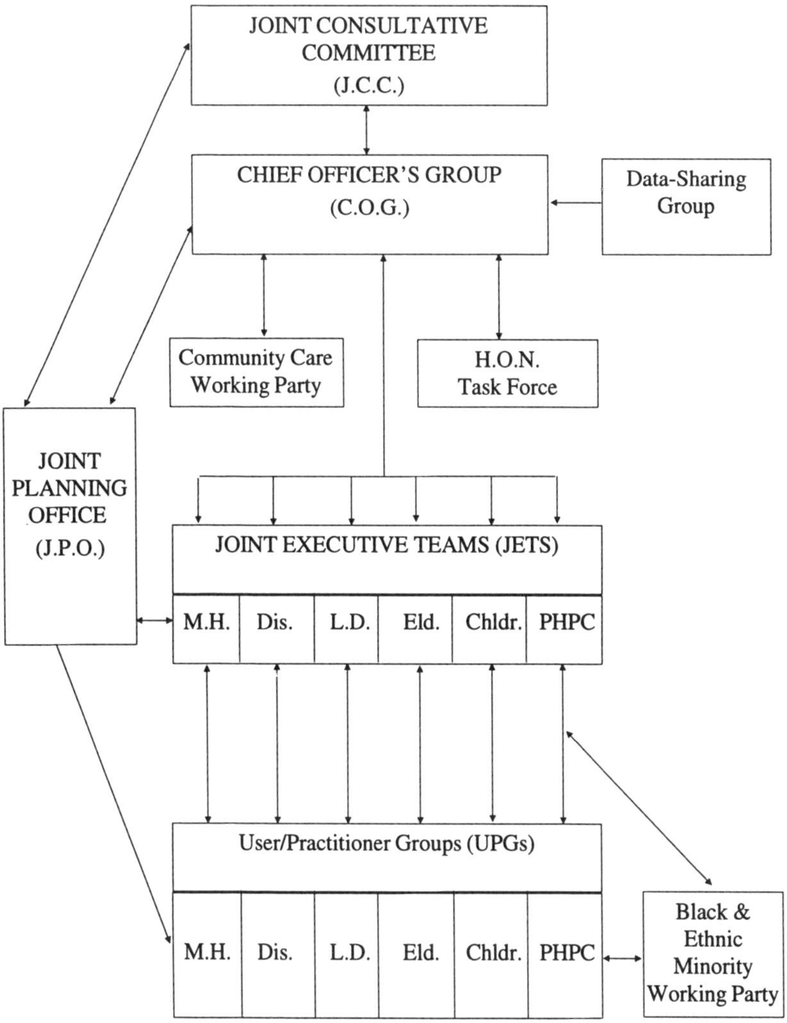

JOINT CONSULTATIVE COMMITTEE (J.C.C.)

CHIEF OFFICER'S GROUP (C.O.G.)

Data-Sharing Group

Community Care Working Party

H.O.N. Task Force

JOINT PLANNING OFFICE (J.P.O.)

JOINT EXECUTIVE TEAMS (JETS)

M.H.	Dis.	L.D.	Eld.	Chldr.	PHPC

User/Practitioner Groups (UPGs)

M.H.	Dis.	L.D.	Eld.	Chldr.	PHPC

Black & Ethnic Minority Working Party

Figure 5 Needs assessment: the four spider model

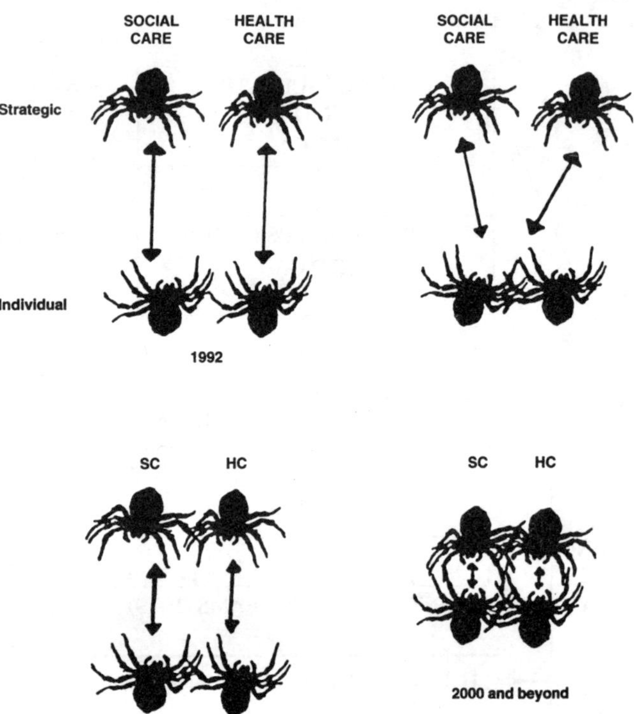

Hackney's present position is the top left hand corner. Health and social services have separate assessment processes both at the strategic level of needs assessment and at the individual assessment of need level. Some legs of the spiders are reaching out and getting entwined. For example, the FHSA is funding research into GP 75+ assessments and community care assessments. But we have a long way to go to the ideal model in the bottom left hand corner, a decade or so on. There has to be vertical and horizontal movement. In particular, the aggregated results of individual assessments of need must influence and affect the strategic needs assessment and subsequent allocation of resources so that there is a closer fit along the vertical. Horizontally, as health and social services jointly commission at the strategic level and jointly assess at the individual level, we get the sideways movement.

Allocation and rationing at the strategic level

Most of what I want to say concerns the individual assessment of need level, as it is my belief that 'Care in the Community in the Next Decade and Beyond' will be made or broken there, not by the speed and sophistication with which we develop our needs-based budgets and ever tighter eligibility criteria.

But let me first give you an idea of how we are allocating and rationing the resources we have or think we have within social services. The policy agreed by Committee is to target those most in need but to retain a balance of services, either in-house or with independent providers, which contribute to maintaining people's independence. So resource centres for elderly people are in, but holidays are out. A higher proportion of the home care budget will be spent on intensive domiciliary care schemes, but the level of shopping and housework will be maintained by delivering it in a cheaper more effective way.

Over the last two years we have top-sliced budgets and created a £350,000 care management budget. Our private and voluntary placements budget stands at £4.5 million. These two budgets plus the majority of the transfer funding will be put together and allocated out across our specialist care management teams using a combination of criteria – Census figures, present spend patterns, known pressure points, desired policy shifts and findings from some sophisticated needs assessment research to which Bobbie Jacobson will be referring. We are devising shadow budgets for our in-house block contracts, in particular home care, and care management teams and hospital teams will have first call. This is crude and very much the start of an interactive process. It was revealing that, although our care management pilots helped people 'think money and priorities', it did not assist in indicating levels of need.

The next step in the rationing process, as I understand it, is setting the eligibility criteria, particularly for those expensive packages of care and nursing homes which could break the budget. I tend to go rather blank at the phrase 'eligibility criteria'. I think it is because I associate it with the rather facile lists senior managers used to send down in my days as a social worker. However, I am encouraged that there is confusion elsewhere as to how best to go about it. One set of guidance we are encouraged to use states emphatically: 'We anticipate that only in very extreme circumstances would an Authority change its eligibility criteria in mid year'. Another organisation we looked to for support says: 'It is essential to have at least monthly checks of actual and estimated numbers so that if the gap is too wide, the criteria can be tightened or loosened'.

As my members make it very clear to me that not overspending the budget is number one priority, the second piece of advice seems more realistic at this stage. We are devising what I call the Social Fund method of rationing. We will work out how many complex packages and/or residential and nursing home places we can afford to buy and we will allocate so much money per month throughout the year. Frontline staff in health and social services will be involved in deciding who will get what and when, following their assessment, if demand outstrips the funding. Once the monthly upper limit figure is reached people will have to wait or be given less than they need. Only reluctantly will money and resources, be shifted from people not under the care management system, i.e. those deemed to have less pressing needs. Some health colleagues on the provider side are, I think, just realising that their presently blocked beds are not going to be miraculously emptied, but most recognise that it is in all our interests to maintain a balance of care.

The context and process of assessment of need

Let me return to the individual assessments. The aggregation of findings from them will eventually turn the allocation process I have just described into a more sophisticated process. It should also direct us towards more effective service contracts – ones which users really want. How our staff carry out these assessments is therefore a vital link in the chain. I would contend that the process is more 'art' than 'science'.

My other contention is that to make sense of an individual's problems in a way that will result in creative packages of care, you have to take account of the whole social situation and make use of what it has to offer. This will do as much for making the money go further as contracts with major providers – a process of 'Networks before Contracts'.

The context

The Hackney context for these assessments is shown on Figure 6.

Figure 6 The context of assessment

Levels of Assessment | **Eligibility**

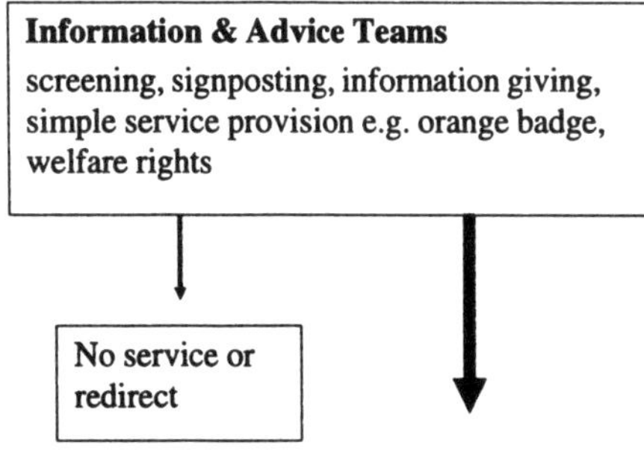

* available to all on open access basis
* good information will ensure appropriate referrals

Community Care Teams
Initial assessment of individuals
Named worker service to GPs
Creating and maintaining community support systems

Service providers

* available on appointment basis only to those individuals who have a need not satisfied by I&A service and whose need seems to be one which social services can satisfy
* emergencies will be dealt with when they arise
* resources prioritised to people facing unacceptable risks, risk of losing independence and where carer support needs maintaining
* as resources allow we can work with people to improve the quality of their lives

Assessment & care management teams

Elderly x 4
Sensory Imp.
Learning Diff.
Drugs & Alcohol
Mental Health
Physical Disab.
HIV/ AIDS

* available for individuals who are on the threshold of residential or nursing home care or whose needs are so complex or specialised that the services they require need a care management approach, i.e. expensive

N.B. The Hospital Teams will work in a similar way to the Community Care Teams incorporating the role of Information & Advice staff.

In each of our four areas we will have an information and advice team, a community care team and a care management team for elderly people under an area community care manager working to the assistant director – the elderly and community purchasing arm. There is a special needs and hospital purchasing arm with a special needs manager managing the specialist care management teams and the hospital teams. Hospital social work teams will do the full range of assessments and have a clear discharge function but will not hold care management budgets. Mental health purchasing is rather separate in the management structure at the moment as we await the outcome of discussions on community mental health teams.

Information and advice teams

The key tasks of these teams are :

1. Information giving
2. Money advice
3. Screening and redirection
4. Making appointments for assessments by the community care team

The information and advice teams will be open to all. They will not be undertaking any of the covert rationing with which we are all familiar – rotten reception areas and telephones never answered. All our offices are scheduled for refurbishment and we run a six-monthly quality check on telephone-answering. Good information will be a key to assisting users to opt in or out themselves and to reach realistic expectations of what is on offer. Some staff, I have learnt, are worried that information will open floodgates of demand, so we have a training task there. We are some way off getting comprehensive information coverage, but there are one or two excellent inroads.

Community care teams

The key tasks of these teams are:

1. Initial assessments of all adult users leading either to a simple service arrangement or a referral to a specialist care management team.
2. Liaison with primary and community health colleagues including a named worker contact for GPs.

3. Creating and maintaining community support systems – I will come back to this.

Assessments will be by appointment only unless it is a crisis and will be for those people who appear to have a need which could be satisfied by the department. The eligibility criteria for assessment is deliberately broad with a top priority of unacceptable risk down a continuum to quality of life. Local managers are expected to make professional judgements as to how assessment time is allocated taking account of these priorities and given their resources, local circumstances and skills available. I realise professional judgement is not a very popular concept these days, but I do believe they know better than head office managers how best to ration and allocate resources within broad policy parameters. They will be shifting resources as best they can to ensure a steady, safe, reliable service and assessment appointments will be made bearing in mind the broad priorities. We have to remember, however, that dealing with human beings is a messy, complex and skilled occupation and those trained staff at the frontline need to be allowed to use their ingenuity to deliver a good assessment and care service.

Let me elaborate on the task of creating and maintaining community support systems – 'Networks before Contracts'. This for me is the context within which assessments and service provision ought to take place if we are going to recapture the excitement and commitment generated by the Griffiths Report (and Barclay some years before) for the provision of care in the community through informal networks. If we ignore this context, we are in danger of leaving our frontline staff alienated and disillusioned, thinking that their jobs are only about unblocking hospital beds and filling up those in independent nursing homes. We will also miss the opportunity to create and make use of the informal care we need if we are going to give people what they want and the cheap care we need if we are going to make our dwindling resources go further.

We must all be aware that a great deal of research shows that a high proportion of elderly people enter residential care at a point of crisis because their informal networks have broken down – a carer being taken ill or neighbours being rehoused. Hurried temporary admission to residential care, more often than not, ends up as permanent care. We could now use our purchasing budgets to buy in flexible care which could fill the gaps left by relatives and friends, or we could 'enable' the community to provide its own caring networks. There is nothing new in this type of work, but I want to ensure that Hackney's community care structure encourages it to happen. The community care teams will be given some money to develop this way of working and I will expect to see developed such things as neighbourhood care schemes, Sunday lunch clubs provided by the local pub, or the church group helped to focus their energies into training as bereavement counsellors.

I am not of course saying that all residential care can be prevented by creating these informal community support services, or that all people's needs can be satisfied without resort to expensive professional care. But even two residential places prevented by a neighbourhood care scheme stepping into the breach covers the cost of a worker undertaking this kind of work. It makes economic sense and can certainly have a great impact on improving people's quality of life, so allowing us to loosen the eligibility criteria.

The process of assessment and rationing

I want to make a final point about the actual process of assessing an individual's needs and how rationing may operate at that level. I was at a conference last week where Professor Olive Stevenson was talking about her latest piece of research undertaken with Phyllida Parsloe (Stevenson and Parsloe, 1993). They have interviewed social workers and occupational therapists about their 'burning issues'. One recurring theme was concern that an assessment, in the brave new community care world, was seen as only a short, time-limited mechanistic process, when anyone who does the work knows it can be a long drawn-out, uncertain process. A second theme was 'Will I have to stop using my counselling skills if I am a care manager?' To which our answer must be 'No', if under the heading of counselling we include empathy, respect, acceptance, listening and understanding. These must surely be part of the care manager's armoury along with the skills of negotiation, challenging, cajoling, persuasion, conceptualising and problem-solving. A book called *Empowerment, Assessment, Care Management and the Skilled Worker* expands on these skills(Smale and Tuson, 1993).

Without these skills, successful assessments of people's complex problems will not be possible. And, by successful, I mean a process which recognises the expertise of the user and carer in assessing their own needs, which takes account of the social situation, which is open and exploratory and which results in a negotiated settlement between user and worker and an understanding of who is doing what, for whom, when and how much it will cost.

This process is very different from one which relies on the worker asking questions and gathering information to see if the user fits or meets certain criteria that will make them eligible for services – the tick box or 'scientific' approach to assessment.

In Hackney, we will be struggling towards the negotiated settlement form of assessment and we will be training our staff (and trying to control our computers) to allow this 'art' form to develop. Rationing is an integral part of the process rather than a series of neatly imposed cut-off points. If funds get low, people in our highest priority brackets may not get everything they need, but they will be involved in deciding what they will and will not have rather than having a rationed package offered to them. It is my strong belief that people in Hackney are actually rather better at rationing and understanding the ways of making a little go a long way than we are. We would be foolish not to involve them.

In summary, Hackney will be training its staff to be skilled assessors. They will need their old but refined social work skills along with negotiation and problem-solving skills. They will be expected to wheel and deal and facilitate community resources as a way of delivering what people want and making the money stretch further. There is of course a limit to how far the money will stretch no matter how inventive and entrepreneurial we are. In the end tightening the eligibility criteria will mean taking more risks as people remain at home with lower levels of service.

Needs assessment and rationing in health care at the population level (Bobbie Jacobson)

A marriage between assessing individual health and social needs and population needs must finally be made on earth, and not elsewhere. The health authorities and social services have no illusions about the difficulties we face ahead in making choices that might be good for the population and not some individuals. This has not prevented us from proceeding together to conduct joint needs assessment work. We believe the rest will follow.

The differences between a public health perspective on assessment of need and assessing individual need for care can be inferred from Figures 7 and 8, where the emphasis is clearly on the population, and on interventions that are effective.

Figure 7 Needs assessment: the public health role

- focus on key priorities
- emphasis on whole population, not selected users
- includes assessment of effectiveness of services
- services required may be outside traditional DHA control
- involves user/public input
- requires a local orientation to national research
- includes economic appraisal where possible

Figure 8 What is health need?

Need for health

- "A State of complete *physical, mental and social* well-being" (WHO)

Relative need for health

- Hips, heart or housing?

Need for health care (local)

- Informal, primary, secondary etc.

Need for social, environmental, housing, leisure services etc. (local)

Need for government resources, policy, action (national)

Clearly, conflict arises when community perceptions of need differ from those of professionals or from systematically analysed need. Figure 9 illustrates this point by summarising the differences in rankings of the health and social interventions found in a recent study we did comparing priority needs expressed by a random sample of the local Hackney community with those of groups of Hackney professionals.

Figure 9 Main results of a public priorities survey in City and Hackney, 1992

Services/treatments	Public	GPs	Consultants	Public health doctors
Treatments for children with life threatening illness (eg leukaemia)	1	5	2	9
Special care and pain relief for people who are dying (eg hospice care)	2	4	4	8
Medical research for new treatments	3	11	8	11
High technology surgery and procedures which treat life threatening conditions (eg heart/liver transplants)	4	12	12	12
Preventive services (eg screening, immunisation)	5	6	7	4
Surgery to help people with disabilities to carry out everyday tasks (eg hip replacements)	6	8	5	5 equal
Therapy to help people with disabilities to carry out everyday tasks (eg speech therapy, physio-therapy, occupational therapy)	7	7	10	5 equal
Services for people with mental illness (eg psychiatric wards, community psychiatric nurses)	8	2	1	1 equal
Intensive care for premature babies who weigh less than 1½lbs and are unlikely to survive	9	13	13	15 equal
Long stay care (eg hospital and nursing home for the elderly)	10	3	6	10
Community services/care at home (eg district nurses)	11	1	3	1 equal
Health education services (eg campaigns encouraging people to lead healthy lifestyles)	12	10	11	5 equal
Family planning services (eg contraception)	13	9	9	1 equal
Treatments for infertility (eg test tube babies)	14	14	14	15 equal
Complementary/alternative medicine (eg acupuncture, homeopathy, herbalism)	15	15	16	13 equal
Cosmetic surgery, (eg tattoo removal, removal of disfiguring lumps and bumps)	16	16	15	13 equal
Number of respondents	*322-335*	*63-66*	*112-116*	*4-6**

* Little can be construed from this sample as the numbers were very small

However, public health does have the tools to bring user perceptions into its needs assessment work. A jointly funded study on health and social needs of elderly people, conducted systematically in Hackney, was clearly able to show not only levels of disability in the population, but also user perceptions of unmet need for health and social services (see Figures 10-12). We now know in Hackney that levels of unmet need for chiropody services are greatest, and that resources in future also need to be directed towards the mildly disabled (Figures 11-12).

Figure 10 Needs assessment: an example

Objective

- Promoting independent living in the community in old age

Tools

- Epidemiology, social survey, perceived need

Question

- What percentage of 'elderly' people living in the district are physically disabled?

Estimated total population	
Aged 65-84	22,500
Aged 85+	2,167
Total 65+	24,667

	Mild disability		Moderate disability		Severe disability	
	No.	%	No.	%	No.	%
65-84	15,395	68	4,725	21	2,388	11
85+	555	26	735	34	878	40
All (65+)	15,950	65	5,460	22	3,266	13

Figure 11 Needs assessment: health in old age

District nurse

Category of disability	% with met need
Mild disability	82
Moderate disability	92
Severe disability	89

Foot care/chiropody	
All disability categories	78

Figure 12 Needs assessment: health in old age

Question

- What is the current met/unmet need for specific health and social services?

Home help

Category of disability/dependence (All aged 65+)	% of people whose need is met
Mild disability	82
Moderate disability	89
Severe disability	90

Concluding comments

Clearly, there are no simple solutions to the conflict inherent in meeting both individual and population needs when resources are finite. We believe we have taken a step forward in Hackney by showing our determination to work together, making any differences explicit so that they become easier to resolve in future.

References

Smale, G. and Tuson, G. (1993), *Empowerment, Assessment, Care Management and the Skilled Worker,* HMSO.

Stevenson, D. and Parsloe, P. (1993) *Community Care and Empowerment,* Joseph Rowntree Foundation.

Rationing: a Philosophy of Care

Terry Bamford
Executive Director of Housing and Social Services
Royal Borough of Kensington and Chelsea

The inevitability of rationing has been highlighted by the previous papers, which have focused on ways in which rationing can be made more rational and more responsive to the needs of users. The task of deciding who gets what, when and in what volume remains constant as managers struggle to find ways of allocating scarce goods and resources.

How these rationing decisions are reached is at the heart of current debate. In common with health care, social services are being obliged to become more explicit about their rationing criteria. In health, these decisions are headline material, when heroic surgery saves a life or dying patients go untreated. It is rarely so eye-catching in social care. A reduction in home-help hours, longer waits for occupational therapy assessments and delays in admission to residential homes are less dramatic, but they too represent the fruits of resource decisions, which have given to some while placing increased burdens on others. Decisions of such critical importance in people's lives require sound philosophical underpinning. Pragmatism is not enough, and too often semantic confusion is the order of the day.

Need is the watchword of the 1990s. The new world of Community Care is as unequivocal as the Children Act. Need is the determinant. Local authorities have drawn up long lists of categories of children in need under the Children Act. They are currently engaged in spelling out the criteria to be applied to assessments under the NHS and Community Care Act. Value statements, however, are difficult to discern, hidden away behind the veil of the woolly generalisations about those most in need, those requiring complex assessments, people with multiple needs and so on. Need can be the user's view of need (felt need), the user's expressed need experienced in demand for services, or the professional's view of assessed need. The Community Care Guidance implicitly acknowledges that hitherto these professional views of need have been conditioned by available resources, and the switch from service and resource-led assessment to need-based assessment is at the heart of the new culture.

The language of Government guidance requires us to target resources at those most in need. Targeting as a word carries with it the smack of efficiency. Its clear implication is that untargeted services are wasteful and poorly-managed. In social care, services have always been targeted. Personal and social services have never achieved the universal status of other welfare provision. The stigma which has accompanied some welfare services since the days of the Poor Law has not wholly been eroded. Establishing eligibility for services requires more than proof of citizenship. It requires demonstrable need. When, therefore, *Caring For People* says 'in future the Government will encourage the targeting of home-based services on those people whose need for them is greatest', an alternative formulation might be 'in future, the Government will encourage the limitation of home-based services to people who are at the margin of residential or nursing home care'. Targeting is rationing, dressed up in more acceptable language.

The very word rationing, of course, brings back folk memories of queuing and ration books. The very concept of the ration book was based on equality, on an equal allocation of scarce goods to all. I want to look, not at the three Es: Economy, Effectiveness and Efficiency of the Audit Commission, but at five Es: Equality, Equity, Efficiency, Effectiveness and Entitlement. By looking at these five Es and testing them against concepts of rights, needs and fairness, one can begin to identify a conceptual basis for rationing in social care.

I want to use Mrs Smith, Mrs Jones and Mr Brown to test out the help which the five E's provide in providing a basis for a philosophy of care. All are elderly. The task of rationing resources across client groups raises a different set of issues.

Mrs Smith is 89 years old, living alone, depressed and disabled by arthritis. She has few social contacts other than her daily home help and meal service. Her daughter lives 80 miles away and wants her to go into a home.

Mrs Jones is 78, quite active despite a recent fall. She lives at the top of a 4-storey block without a lift, struggles with the steps. She gets home help twice a week, but no meal service. She goes to a day centre a couple of times each week. Her daughter calls daily.

Mr Brown is 67. His wife died last year. Physically fit but depressed, he is drinking too much, his flat is messy, and his interest in life is limited to the pub and the TV. His GP has referred him for home help assessment.

When it comes to butter and sugar and jam, the ***equality*** of the ration book is legitimate in giving an equal share of scarce goods to all. It is legitimate because it would have offended the egalitarian spirit of post-war days to have exposed such goods to a free market. But when it comes to personal social services, equality is inadequate and inappropriate as a basis for distribution. Providing a home-help service to every adult household with a household member over 65 would both spread a scarce resource so thinly that it would be of little benefit to anybody and would also result in large numbers of people having a service that they did not require. Giving a service in equal volumes to Mrs Smith, Mrs Jones and Mr Brown would not reflect their unequal needs. However, to give a home-help service to every household with a member over the age of 85 would be one way of ensuring what Bleddyn Davies and colleagues call 'horizontal target efficiency', ensuring that the service reaches all those in the eligible group.

Equity means fairness: the sense of justice which is part of us all. It is equity which often dominates public opinion. Scandals occur when people do not get what is regarded as a fair allocation of scarce goods. Selection by ballot may be equitable for the National Lottery or in the USA for exemption from the Draft, but is not regarded as equitable if the decision is one of who has kidney dialysis. Equity is seductive because it contains within it a sense of desert and thus opens the door to subjective preferences being applied by the allocator. Senior managers, however, strive to apply equity in the sense of proportional justice, ensuring that people with similar needs receive similar treatment and similar services. Their bid to do so is often subverted by social workers whose concern for individual justice and securing fair treatment for the client with whom they are working often ignores the opportunity cost for others of increasing the allocation to an individual client.

Equity would dictate that Mrs Smith got a higher volume of service than Mrs Jones, and that both got more than Mr Brown.

The involvement of individual social workers can not only distort considerations of equity, but also affect efficiency. ***Efficiency*** is the maximisation of outputs for a given level of inputs. Maximising efficiency often demands standardisation. Any deviation from the standard solution in pursuit of individual needs represents a diminution from the collective good. If Mrs Smith and Mr Brown lived next door to each other, but Mrs Jones was several miles away and involved travelling time – an efficiency approach to rationing might discard a service to Mrs Jones because of the opportunity cost.

The pursuit of pure utilitarianism – the greatest increase in welfare for the greatest number – is not a sound basis for decision-making in personal social services. It is unsound, first, because of the absence of any clear causal relationship between inputs and outcomes. This is not peculiar to social services. The same is true of much community based health care. Secondly, it ignores the large component in social care, which is social maintenance, which is giving care and support to people whose needs are so great and resources so few that contact and friendship is the only realistic service that one can offer. The debate about the degree to which this is a function of Social Services departments, as opposed to the voluntary sector, and the degree to which social work skills are required in the process remains open, but effectiveness alone is inadequate as a basis for decision-making.

What would be effective for the three elderly clients? A care package may keep Mrs Smith at home for a few months more. Mrs Jones, however, would derive the greatest long-term benefit from care management because more appropriate accommodation would address her primary problem. Mr Brown needs help, but whether it will offer more than contact is doubtful.

Entitlement: do clients have rights? In the value base of social work, there is much emphasis on client self-determination and the rights of clients to be fully involved in decisions about their future. Clients now have a statutory right to choice in relation to residential care. It is a very limited right, constrained firstly by an assessment of need to establish the eligibility threshold, and secondly by the cost limits set on places by the local authority. Choice is part of the new language, but it is rarely more than rhetoric. Choice requires surplus capacity if it is to be real.

Social workers already encourage user participation in decisions often using the rhetoric of user-empowerment, but sometimes little more is involved than a modicum of participation in decision-making. The real choices available to elderly people are in practice, whether or not to accept a service. There is little question of selecting services on a mix-and-match basis. The rhetoric of choice obscures the unacknowledged conflict between user choice and needs-led assessment. As the PSI study on the elderly said 'just feeling tired and lonely and unable to cope at home will no longer secure a place in residential care, even if you are 85' (Allen et al, 1992). Mrs Smith, Mrs Jones and Mr Brown have no entitlements, no enforceable rights to service. Looking for entitlements in social care is a barren exercise Twenty-two years after the Chronically Sick and Disabled Persons Act, there has been no concerted bid to widen local authorities' statutory duties to provide services to meet identified needs.

Of the five Es, Equality, Efficiency, Effectiveness and Entitlement, seem flawed as a basis for shaping rationing criteria. Equity, with the reservations, is the one candidate still standing. It is important then, to address ways in which the tensions that were noted between individual justice and proportional justice can be minimised. Most of the available research material on how scarce resources are allocated is derived from the study of elderly people and their carers. The Equal Opportunities Commission, Policy Studies Institute, the Personal Social Services Research Unit (PSSRU) all point to certain common themes. Households with access to an informal carer receive less than those where there is no carer. (Mrs Jones would probably get less service than her needs dictated.) Elderly men get more help than elderly women. (Mr Brown would get a service.) Those with reservations about Social Services intervention get more home-help support than those who welcome it, presumably on the Avis principle of trying harder.

What checks and balances may we look to? The requirement to publish criteria for assessment and the allocation of services presents a new opportunity to rethink the approach to care. First, it requires departments to render explicit what is often left implicit in decisions about who gets what. Professional discretion will be circumscribed as clients get clear statements about the basis of assessment. Initially, many departments will retreat behind statements at a high level of generality. Resource constraints, if nothing else, will oblige them to be more and more specific in defining eligibility. Secondly, publicity for the assessment criteria brings them into the legitimate arena for public debate. If it can be shown that groups excluded by the eligibility criteria have needs as great or greater than those which are being met, policies will have to be modified. As data builds up from the process of needs assessment, that modification should take place. Being explicit about rationing – while an advance on pragmatism – is not enough.

If there is a genuine desire to establish citizenship rights for the clients of personal social services, the stranglehold of professional discretion on determining eligibility has to be broken. Equity has to be translated into entitlement – a clear, publicly stated and legally enforceable entitlement to a given volume of service with higher levels of dependency matched by higher levels of service volume. Thus Mrs Smith might have an entitlement, possibly even expressed in a cash equivalent voucher to 25 service units, Mrs Jones to 10 and Mr Brown to 5 reflecting their differential dependency. Concepts of entitlement would oblige departments to face up to the ethical dilemma of whether they are willing to pay £50, £60 or £70,000 a year to sustain individual preference for community living at an opportunity cost for other potential beneficiaries.

The other Es – Efficiency, Effectiveness, Equality and Equity – have a part to play in shaping those entitlements, but until clients' rights are buttressed in this way, too much power will rest with professionals.

The new structure of needs-led assessment is about to come into force. There is still time to ensure that this does not become distorted into a further accretion of professional power, but that social work values dictate the development of rights and entitlements, rather than the mirage of choice, for users.

References

Allen, I., Hogg, D. and Peace, S. (1992), *Elderly People: Choice, Participation and Satisfaction,* Policy Studies Institute.

Who Gets What – and Why? Ethical Frameworks for Managers

Jeff Girling
Senior Fellow, Health Services Management Unit
University of Manchester

> It appears to me in ethics as in all other philosophical studies, the difficulties and disagreements, of which its history are full, are mainly due to a very simple cause: namely to the attempt to answer questions, without firstly discovering precisely what question it is which you desire to answer (G.E. Moore (1903), *Principia Ethica*).

In health care the discipline known as 'medical ethics' emerged out of the need by clinicians to reflect on the sort of criteria which they thought ought to govern their professional relationships with their patients or clients. As a result we find the basic language being provided by such key concepts as autonomy, non-maleficence and beneficence.

Whilst managers need to be fully aware of such debates within medical ethics, there is a corresponding need to reflect on the ethical implications of their own specific forms of decision making.

Perhaps this is no clearer than in the debate around rationing. Resource allocation decisions beg answers to the question of not only 'who gets what?', but also 'who gets what – and why?' Managerial decision making is fairly comfortable with the financial dimension, and increasingly with the economic. It is less familiar with the ethical dimension. However, with the creation of the commissioning function within strategic management comes the need for the development of ethical frameworks for managers to help them work through decision making dilemmas. This paper focuses on that issue.

What might be called managerial ethics is still in the early stages of development within health and social care. What is offered here is a contribution to that debate by looking at some of the key ingredients which might be included in a decision making framework. Particular attention is paid to the interplay between utility, rights, and equity and how these might be combined in a helpful way. Indeed, the discussion ends with an outline decision tree which is offered as a way of framing our thinking on issues such as rationing.

Developing a framework

Ethical dilemmas typically take the form of 'what ought I to do?' (in any given situation). For a manager faced with allocating scarce resources – who wants to make sure that this takes place against some sense of fairness – the rationing debate poses the ethical dilemma in a very real sense.

What we need to do is to see whether there are any helpful pointers which can be applied specifically to the managerial context. A helpful starting point might be to start our search with the first principles of ethical reasoning (Beauchamp and Childress, 1983). In this respect an ethical framework consists of theories, principles, rules and actions arranged in some form of relationship with each other. In fact they form a hierarchy. Accordingly, particular actions in particular situations are justified by checking back to rules and principles which derive their justification from ethical theories.

There are two main ethical theories which have dominated ethical reasoning. These are utilitarianism and deontology. The latter (derived from the Greek term for 'duty') is concerned with the actual motive behind an action, not by its consequences. The former however judges the rightness and wrongness of an action purely by its consequences.

There are several types of utilitarianism (Brandt, 1992). However, as a decision-making paradigm it is most familiar to managers faced with the necessity to reconcile the claims of different claimants and the need to get results for their organisations and the users of their services.

This is not to claim that managers endorse an abstract theory and use it as an explicit guide to answering the question 'what ought I to do?' It is more a case of recognising that, if the culture of management is informed by a theoretical tradition at all, then its closest affinity is with utilitarianism. As a point of comparison it may be the case that the clinical culture, on the other hand, is much more comfortable with the deontological concerns of, for example, autonomy, paternalism, and patient confidentiality. This may incidentally account for the apparent fact that managers and clinicians sometimes seem to inhabit different ethical worlds. It will be extremely interesting in the next few years to evaluate the impact of GP fundholding, clinical directorates, and care management upon clinical cultures – especially if these developments lead to a closer involvement in the rationing process. We may well see a greater synergy between the two managerial and clinical cultures as a result.

Of course, as well as lofty principles, any practical framework for managers must also include another key ingredient – namely that of factual beliefs. For example, if we hold that policy X is wrong because it does not lead to any perceivable benefits to those affected, then we have presupposed certain beliefs about the facts of that situation. Many disagreements about the allocation of resources not only turn on basic values and concepts of equity (as they certainly do), but also on factual claims about the expected impact or outcome of the decisions. As a result, an ethical framework for managers has to include ethical principles and considerations of factual outcomes.

Utility, rights and equity

To restate the overall question, the key issue is whether there are any principles and guides which may help the emergence of an ethical approach to the many conundrums and quandaries which are thrown up when needs and demands outstrip the supply of available resources.

In fact, there are three principles which can claim a privileged place in the framework. These are utility, rights, and equity. In terms of a decision making process they might be seen as providing the main conditions to be satisfied. All are necessary for a managerially ethical decision. None of the three is sufficient on its own.

These three concepts cannot claim any self-evident grounds for being afforded the privileged status in the framework. Ethicists have not yet managed to find ultimate justification for ethical principles. However, utility, rights and equity are not arbitrarily chosen. They are chosen because they are consistent with the historical value base of public sector provision of health and social care (HMSO, 1979). Moreover, they are also consistent with the ethos of allocating resources under the conditions of competitive contracts to best meet the needs of service users. In sum, they could be said to be the implied ethical tests of the commissioning arrangements.

Let us take each of these concepts briefly in turn, starting with utility. We have already made the suggestion that management is closest to utilitarianism than other ethical theories. The concept of utility is the central principle of utilitarianism. And for most public sector managers it is perhaps the most familiar (even though they may not always use the term explicitly).

There is certainly a social ethic entailed in the underlying decision-making rule of utilitarianism, namely that decisions should aim to produce the greatest good for the greatest number of stakeholders. It is also possible to see how this principle of utility *per se*, i.e. maximising benefits over costs, is very close to the hearts of managers operating within tight cash limits.

So there is little doubt that the starting point for a managerialist ethic has to be rooted somewhere in the concept of utility. It is here that ethical reasoning and factual belief come together, for it is a feature of the utilitarian approach that decisions are judged by their likely outcomes. This in turn entails that those consequences can somehow be measured and that judgements can be made between competing options. That basis is usually cast in terms of benefits over costs in some form of calculus. For some, this might be the end of the line as far as ethical decision making goes. However there are still two other ingredients to consider.

Rights and equity may be more austere and less 'streetwise' than utility, but rights and equity are important control concepts over the possible excesses of utility. Rights, for example, have been said to be 'trumps over utility' (Plant, 1989).

Certainly, any feasible managerial framework has to be placed in some form of social context, and rights language is especially embedded in the liberal-democratic tradition which is pervasive in our society. From Hobbes and Locke to the present day, theorists have employed the language of rights to make their moral/social arguments (Macedo, 1990). Moreover, our Anglo-American legal tradition is rooted in this tradition.

The key point about rights is that they are enforceable claims which individuals make upon others. However, Plant points out that there is no enforceable claim to a scarce resource (Plant, 1989). It is hard to win the case for a *positive* right to scarce resources. Managers cannot necessarily meet the claim that they ought to satisfy all positive rights, since the sheer fact of scarcity makes it impossible both in principle and in practice. This means that rights have to be seen very much in terms of basic right to *equal consideration* of any claims to resources. In terms of rationing it means an equal access to the decision making mechanisms.

This brings us to our third and final category, namely equity. As a term 'equity' is best seen as synonymous with 'fairness', and in terms of the rationing debate it is best seen as equal access to services on the basis of equal need. It can function as a very powerful substantive concept in discussions around the allocation and distribution of resources. However, for the purposes of the managerial decision making framework, the term 'equity' is best seen in terms of procedural justice. What this means in practice is the development of explicit groundrules to govern our decision making and the insistence on clear and consistent rules which spell out which criteria are relevant and which are not. Once this has happened then all parties can be clear about the relevant grounds for a decision.

In this way equity (procedural justice) lies in the pursuit of an even-handed discharge of due process based on an equal treatment within relevant criteria. For the purposes of the ethical framework for managers those criteria are focused on the adjudication between competing claims to maximise utility, together with a respect for the rights of the competitors for the scarce resources. Other considerations are not permitted on the grounds that they are not relevant to the task of making an ethically based decision over 'who gets what?'

The decision tree

From this brief look at utility, rights and equity, we have now covered the main ingredients of the framework. We can conclude by seeing these in the form of a decision tree in order to illustrate the ethical decision making process. We can do this by way of a hypothetical case study.

Suppose that the joint health and social services commissioning team want to review a key aspect in the provision of mental health services. They have identified two broad options – one for a new facility on the site of the general hospital – the other proposal being for the development of a community mental health centre. Let us suppose that they are both subjected to some form of feasibility study

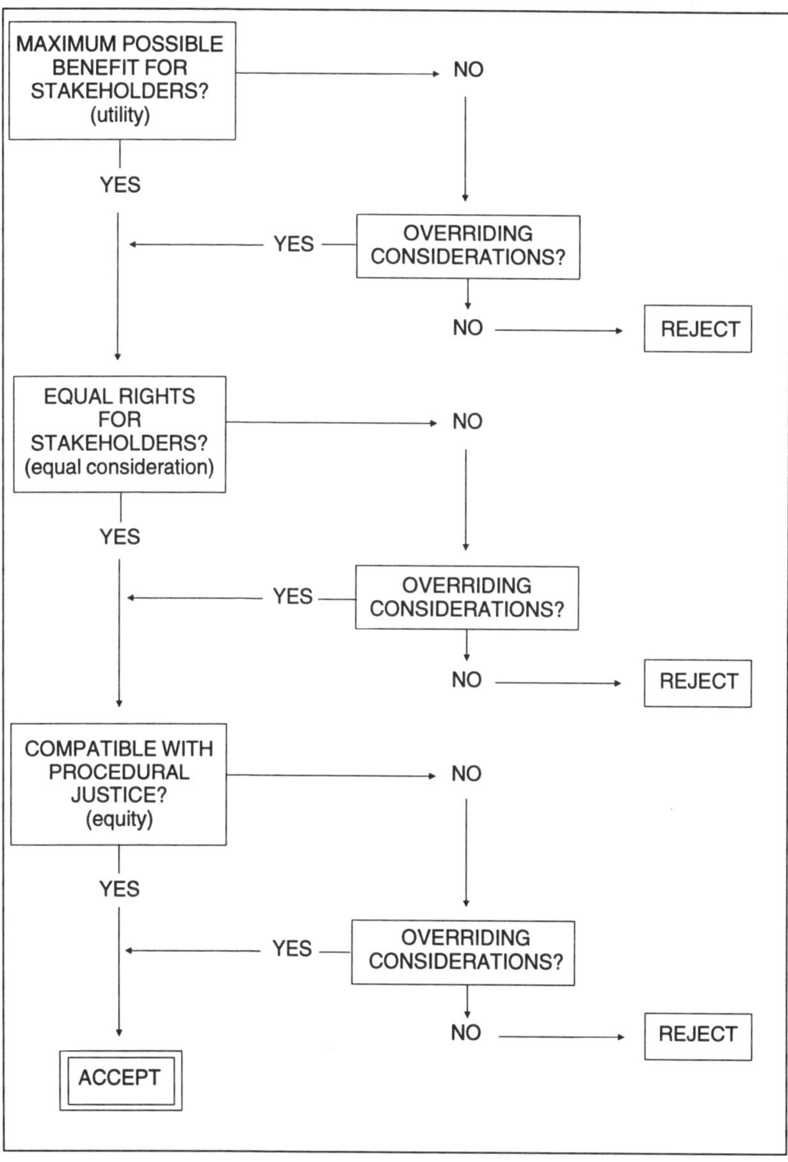

and option appraisal. This option appraisal reaches the conclusion that the two proposals would each produce equal benefits (value for money, health gain, user views, etc). However, let us suppose that one of the proposals (A) is strongly lobbied for by its sponsors, whereas the other proposal (B) does not receive the same form of proactive backing. As a result the commissioning team find themselves funding proposal A. The question then is this: how would that decision be judged by our ethical framework?

Testing the decision

The first stage concerns the test of utility. Obviously it turned out that stakeholders represented by proposal A achieved maximum possible benefit from the process. However, in the facts of our hypothetical case there is no problem here. The outcome was not sub-optimal since we can recall that both proposals were judged to score the same in the option appraisal. The second test looks at the question of rights. Here again it would seem that the commissioning team's decision would pass the test of the ethical framework. There is no evidence of a violation of positive or procedural rights here. As events turned out the sponsors of proposal B chose not to exercise the opportunity to point out proactively what they saw as the particular strengths of their option. However, the open lobbying by supporters of proposal A meant that there was no deceit. It could be argued (legitimately) that voluntary inaction implies consent to the action of the other party.

It is in fact on the issue of equity that an ethicist might say that A's position is suspect. Justice would have been served if there had been a clear and relevant difference between A's and B's proposals. However, the option appraisal found them to be equivalent in terms of their respective benefits and respective utility scores. However, A's actions fall foul on the equity front on the grounds that the lobbying served to create ethically irrelevant differences between A and B. This would therefore result in an ethically sub-optimal decision. The only relevant criteria which ought to count in the framework are those of utility and respect for equal rights.

As a result of using this ethical decision tree, the commissioners would not have made their decision to fund A on justified grounds. They might well have stuck with it, but it could be held that it would be ethically flawed within the framework outlined here.

Conclusions

So, there are a number of ways in which decisions can be made, and the ethical decision tree is presented as a procedural model for consideration. It may well be that, in the illustration, the blocking of proposal A on the grounds of breach of procedural justice strikes us as rather unlikely. It just would not happen that way. Maybe. However it is suggested that the value of the approach is as an overall framework which addresses the need to see ethical criteria as serious criteria for making decisions over the allocation of resources. The history of decision making in health and social services provides ample proof of allocative decisions being made on non-ethical grounds. Witness the grounds by which medical technology is often funded as a result of lobbying by powerful groups rather than on clearly assessed and evaluated need. Such decisions result not only in unfair outcomes, but also result in the inefficient use of resources. This is where – through the concept of opportunity costs – economists and ethicists come together. Under conditions of scarcity, the inefficient use of resources is also unethical.

In conclusion, decisions do have to be made. It is a question of which criteria will guide them. As G.E. Moore says, it all depends on 'what question it is which you desire to answer'.

References

Beauchamp, T. and Childress, J. (1983), *Principles of Biomedical Ethics*, Oxford University Press.

Brandt, R. (1992), *Morality, Utilitarianism and Rights*, Cambridge University Press.

Macedo, S. (1990), *Liberal Virtues*, Oxford University Press.

Moore, G.E. (1903), *Principia Ethica*, Cambridge University Press.

Plant, R. (1989), *Can there be a Right to Health Care?*, Occasional Paper, Institute for Health Policy Studies, University of Southampton.

Royal Commission on the NHS (the Merrison Report) (1979), HMSO.